HIGH FIBER VEGETARIAN COOKBOOK

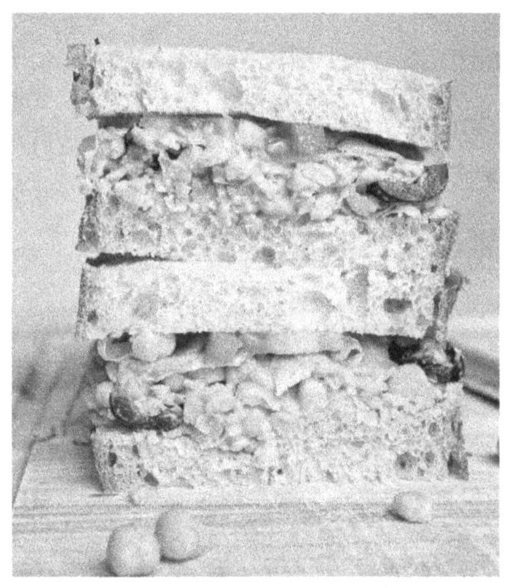

"80 Delicious Plant-Based Recipes for Gut Health and Enhancing Well-Being"

Dayna G. Murphy

Gain Access to Other Titles by the Author:

Table of Content

INTRODUCTION

Lisa, Tom, and Maya, three friends from a small town, decided to start on a high-fiber vegetarian journey together. Lisa, a busy parent, discovered new energy and harmony in her life through vivid salads and fiber-rich fruits. Tom, a fitness enthusiast, realized that increasing his intake of beans and whole grains powered his exercises and improved muscle recovery. High-fiber meals provided sustained focus and helped Maya, a student with a hectic schedule, stay aware during long study sessions. The trio not only enjoyed delicious meals, but they also saw improvements in their overall health. Their high-fiber vegetarian experience became a shared joy, enhancing their life in more ways than one, with laughter shared over lentil soups and avocado toasts.

CHAPTER 1

About High Fiber Diets

A high fiber diet has a lot of dietary fiber, which is a form of carbohydrate found in plant-based foods. Dietary fiber is classified into two types: soluble and insoluble.

1. Fiber that is soluble in water:

- Foods that include it include oats, barley, beans, lentils, fruits, and vegetables.
- with the digestive tract, it dissolves with water to form a gel-like material.
- Lowers cholesterol, stabilizes blood sugar, and promotes a sensation of fullness.

2. Fiber that is insoluble:

- Whole grains, nuts, seeds, and the skins of fruits and vegetables all contain it.
- Although it does not dissolve in water, it adds weight to the feces.

- Prevents constipation and encourages regular bowel motions.

The Advantages of a High Fiber Diet:

- **Digestive Health**: Fiber gives weight to the stool, avoiding constipation and encouraging regular bowel motions.

- **Weight Control**: High fiber foods are frequently lower in calories and create a feeling of fullness, which aids in weight management.

- **Heart Health**: Soluble fiber may help lower cholesterol levels, lowering the risk of heart disease.

- **Blood Sugar Control**: Fiber slows sugar absorption, which aids with blood sugar management.

- **Colon Health:** By fostering a healthy digestive tract, insoluble fiber may help minimize the incidence of colorectal cancer.

A High Fiber Diet Must Include:

- **Whole Grains**: Brown rice, quinoa, whole wheat, and barley are examples of whole grains.
- **Legumes**: Beans, lentils, and chickpeas are examples of legumes.
- **Fruits**: Berries, apples, pears, and oranges are examples of fruits.
- **Vegetables**: Broccoli, carrots, kale, and Brussels sprouts are among the vegetables.
- **Nuts and Seeds**: Almonds, chia seeds, and flaxseeds are examples of nuts and seeds.

It's crucial to remember that increasing fiber consumption should be done gradually, with plenty of water, and matched to individual dietary needs. Before making significant dietary changes, always consult with a healthcare practitioner or a qualified nutritionist.

Benefits of a Vegetarian Lifestyle

Adopting a vegetarian diet, which entails avoiding meat and, in many cases, other animal products, can have a number of health, environmental, and ethical advantages. Here are some significant characteristics of the advantages of a vegetarian lifestyle:

1. Heart Health Improvement:

- Lower levels of saturated fats and cholesterol are generally connected with vegetarian diets, contributing to a lower risk of heart disease.
- Consumption of fruits, vegetables, whole grains, and legumes increases consumption of important nutrients that support cardiovascular health.

2. Weight Control:

- Vegetarian diets are lower in calories and saturated fats, making them ideal for weight control and loss.
- Plant-based foods with high fiber content contribute to a sensation of fullness, lowering the chance of overeating.

3. Reduced Risk of Specific Cancers:

- Some research suggests that a vegetarian diet may reduce the risk of certain cancers, particularly colon cancer.

4. Diabetes Type 2 Prevention and Management:

- Plant-based diets high in whole grains, fruits, and vegetables may help with blood sugar control and lowering the risk of developing type 2 diabetes.

5. Better Digestive Health:

- Plant-based meals' fiber content aids healthy digestion and regular bowel movements, lowering the risk of constipation and other digestive disorders.

6. Environmental Longevity:

- Plant-based foods demand fewer resources, such as land, water, and energy, than rearing livestock for meat production.

- A vegetarian diet can help to minimize greenhouse gas emissions and leave a smaller environmental imprint.

7. Considerations for Ethical Behavior:

- Many people become vegetarians for ethical grounds, such as concerns about animal suffering and the environmental impact of factory farming.

- Choosing plant-based alternatives is consistent with a humane attitude toward animals.

8. Kidney Function Enhancement:

- Plant-based diets may benefit kidney function by reducing acid load on the kidneys as compared to animal protein-rich diets.

9. Anti-Inflammatory Advantages:

- Fruits, vegetables, and nuts are high in antioxidants and anti-inflammatory chemicals, which may help to reduce inflammation in the body.

10. Longevity:

- According to certain research, following a vegetarian diet may be related with enhanced longevity, while many factors contribute to general health and lifespan.

Key Ingredients for High Fiber Cooking

Creating high-fiber meals involves incorporating a variety of plant-based ingredients into your diet. Here are key ingredients that are rich in fiber and can be used for high-fiber cooking:

1. Whole Grains:

- Brown rice
- Quinoa
- Whole wheat pasta
- Barley
- Oats

2. Legumes:

- Lentils
- Chickpeas
- Black beans
- Kidney beans
- Pinto beans

3. Fruits:

- Berries (strawberries, blueberries, raspberries)
- Apples (with skin)

- Pears (with skin)

- Bananas

- Oranges

4. Vegetables:

- Broccoli

- Brussels sprouts

- Carrots

- Spinach

- Kale

- Cauliflower

- Sweet potatoes

5. Nuts and Seeds:

- Almonds

- Chia seeds

- Flaxseeds

- Sunflower seeds

- Pumpkin seeds

6. Whole Grain Bread and Cereals:

- Choose bread and cereals that are made from whole grains to increase fiber content.

7. Root Vegetables:

- Beets

- Turnips

- Rutabagas

- Radishes

8. Legume-based Products:

- Tofu

- Tempeh

- Edamame

9. High-Fiber Snacks:

- Popcorn (air-popped, without excessive butter or oil)

- Whole fruit (with skin)

- Vegetable sticks with hummus

10. Psyllium Husk:

- Psyllium husk is a plant-based source of soluble fiber often used as a supplement or added to recipes to increase fiber content.

11. Seitan:

- Seitan is a high-protein meat substitute made from gluten, and it can be a good source of fiber as well.

12. Whole Grain Flour:

- When baking, consider using whole grain flours like whole wheat flour instead of refined flours.

13. Dried Fruits:

- Dried fruits such as raisins, apricots, and prunes can be added to dishes or eaten as snacks.

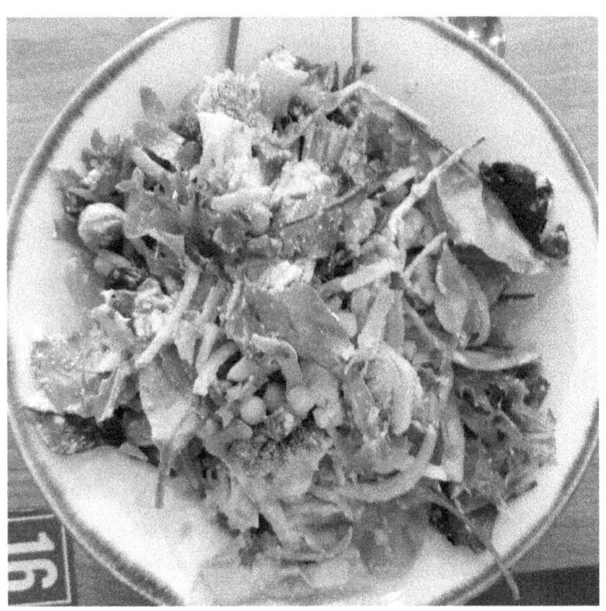

CHAPTER 2

Breakfast Delights

1. Chia Seed Pudding Parfait

Ingredients:

- 3 tablespoons chia seeds
- 1 cup almond milk
- 1 tablespoon maple syrup
- 1/2 cup mixed berries
- 1/4 cup granola
- Sliced almonds for garnish

Instructions:

1. In a jar, mix chia seeds, almond milk, and maple syrup. Stir well and refrigerate overnight.

2. In the morning, layer chia pudding with mixed berries and granola in a glass.

3. Top with sliced almonds.

Prep Time: 5 minutes (plus overnight soaking)

2. Greek Yogurt and Berry Parfait

Ingredients:

- 1 cup Greek yogurt
- 1/2 cup mixed berries (strawberries, blueberries, raspberries)
- 2 tablespoons honey
- 1/4 cup high-fiber cereal
- Chopped mint leaves for garnish

Instructions:

1. In a glass, layer Greek yogurt with mixed berries.

2. Drizzle honey over the layers and top with high-fiber cereal.

3. Garnish with chopped mint leaves.

Prep Time: 5 minutes

3. Spinach and Feta Breakfast Wrap

Ingredients:

- 1 whole grain tortilla
- 2 eggs, scrambled
- Handful of fresh spinach
- 2 tablespoons feta cheese, crumbled
- Salsa for serving

Instructions:

1. Place the tortilla on a flat surface.

2. Layer the scrambled eggs, fresh spinach, and crumbled feta in the center.

3. Roll up the tortilla and serve with salsa.

Prep Time: 10 minutes

4. Banana Walnut Overnight Oats

Ingredients:

- 1/2 cup rolled oats
- 1/2 cup almond milk
- 1 ripe banana, mashed
- 1 tablespoon chopped walnuts
- 1/2 teaspoon cinnamon

Instructions:

1. In a jar, combine rolled oats, almond milk, mashed banana, chopped walnuts, and cinnamon.

2. Mix well, cover, and refrigerate overnight.

3. In the morning, stir and enjoy.

Prep Time: 5 minutes (plus overnight soaking)

5. Veggie Breakfast Burrito

Ingredients:

- 1 whole grain tortilla
- 1/2 cup black beans, cooked
- 1/4 cup diced bell peppers
- 2 tablespoons salsa
- 1/4 cup shredded cheese (cheddar or your choice)

Instructions:

1. Warm the tortilla.

2. Layer black beans, diced bell peppers, salsa, and shredded cheese.

3. Roll up the tortilla and serve.

Prep Time: 10 minutes

6. Peanut Butter Banana Toast

Ingredients:

- 1 slice whole grain bread
- 2 tablespoons peanut butter
- 1 banana, sliced
- Drizzle of honey (optional)

Instructions:

1. Toast the whole grain bread.

2. Spread peanut butter on the toast.

3. Arrange banana slices on top and drizzle with honey if desired.

Prep Time: 5 minutes

7. Berry and Kale Smoothie

Ingredients:

- 1 cup kale, stems removed
- 1/2 cup frozen mixed berries
- 1/2 banana
- 1 cup almond milk
- 1 tablespoon chia seeds

Instructions:

1. Blend kale, mixed berries, banana, almond milk, and chia seeds until smooth.

2. Pour into a glass and enjoy.

Prep Time: 5 minutes

8. Apple Cinnamon Quinoa Bowl

Ingredients:

- 1/2 cup cooked quinoa

- 1 apple, diced
- 1 tablespoon almond butter
- 1/2 teaspoon cinnamon
- 1 tablespoon chopped pecans

Instructions:

1. In a bowl, mix cooked quinoa, diced apple, almond butter, and cinnamon.

2. Top with chopped pecans and serve.

Prep Time: 10 minutes

9. Blueberry Almond Breakfast Cookies

Ingredients:

- 1 cup rolled oats
- 1/2 cup almond flour
- 1/4 cup maple syrup
- 1/4 cup almond butter
- 1/2 teaspoon vanilla extract
- 1/2 cup dried blueberries
- 1/4 cup sliced almonds

Instructions:

1. Preheat the oven to 350°F (175°C).

2. In a bowl, combine rolled oats, almond flour, maple syrup, almond butter, and vanilla extract.

3. Fold in dried blueberries and sliced almonds.

4. Scoop onto a baking sheet and bake for 12-15 minutes until golden.

Prep Time: 15 minutes

10. Mango and Coconut Chia Pudding

Ingredients:

- 3 tablespoons chia seeds
- 1 cup coconut milk
- 1/2 ripe mango, diced
- 1 tablespoon shredded coconut

Instructions:

1. In a jar, mix chia seeds and coconut milk. Stir well and refrigerate for at least 2 hours or overnight.

2. In the morning, layer chia pudding with diced mango in a glass.

3. Top with shredded coconut.

Prep Time: 5 minutes (plus soaking time)

CHAPTER 3

Appetizing Starters

1. Lentil and Vegetable Soup

Ingredients:

- 1 cup dry lentils, rinsed
- 4 cups vegetable broth
- 1 onion, diced
- 2 carrots, chopped
- 2 celery stalks, chopped
- 3 cloves garlic, minced
- 1 teaspoon cumin
- 1 teaspoon paprika
- Salt and pepper to taste
- Fresh parsley for garnish

Instructions:

1. In a large pot, sauté onions, carrots, and celery until softened.

2. Add garlic, cumin, and paprika; cook for another minute.

3. Stir in lentils and vegetable broth. Bring to a boil, then simmer until lentils are tender (about 20-25 minutes).

4. Season with salt and pepper. Garnish with fresh parsley before serving.

Prep Time: 30 minutes

2. Spinach and Artichoke Dip

Ingredients:

- 1 cup frozen spinach, thawed and drained
- 1 can (14 oz) artichoke hearts, drained and chopped
- 1 cup plain Greek yogurt
- 1 cup shredded mozzarella cheese
- 1/2 cup grated Parmesan cheese
- 1 clove garlic, minced
- Salt and pepper to taste
- Whole grain pita or veggie sticks for dipping

Instructions:

1. Preheat the oven to 375°F (190°C).

2. In a bowl, combine spinach, artichoke hearts, Greek yogurt, mozzarella, Parmesan, and garlic.

3. Season with salt and pepper. Transfer to a baking dish.

4. Bake for 20-25 minutes or until bubbly and golden.

5. Serve with whole grain pita or veggie sticks.

Prep Time: 30 minutes

3. Avocado and Black Bean Salsa

Ingredients:

- 1 can (15 oz) black beans, drained and rinsed
- 1 avocado, diced
- 1 cup corn kernels (fresh or frozen, thawed)
- 1/2 red onion, finely chopped
- 1 jalapeño, seeded and diced
- Juice of 2 limes
- Fresh cilantro, chopped
- Salt and pepper to taste
- Tortilla chips for serving

Instructions:

1. In a bowl, combine black beans, diced avocado, corn, red onion, jalapeño, lime juice, and cilantro.

2. Season with salt and pepper. Mix well.

3. Refrigerate for at least 30 minutes before serving.

4. Serve with tortilla chips.

Prep Time: 15 minutes

4. Stuffed Mushrooms with Quinoa and Feta

Ingredients:

- 1/2 large mushrooms, stems removed and chopped
- 1 cup cooked quinoa
- 1/2 cup feta cheese, crumbled
- 2 tablespoons olive oil
- 2 cloves garlic, minced
- Fresh parsley, chopped
- Salt and pepper to taste

Instructions:

1. Preheat the oven to 375°F (190°C).

2. In a skillet, sauté mushroom stems and garlic in olive oil until softened.

3. In a bowl, mix sautéed mixture with cooked quinoa, feta, and fresh parsley.

4. Season with salt and pepper.

5. Stuff each mushroom cap with the quinoa mixture.

6. Bake for 15-20 minutes or until mushrooms are tender.

Prep Time: 30 minutes

5. Baked Zucchini Fritters

Ingredients:

- 2 medium zucchinis, grated and drained
- 1/2 cup whole wheat flour
- 1/4 cup grated Parmesan cheese
- 1 clove garlic, minced
- 1 teaspoon dried oregano
- Salt and pepper to taste
- 2 eggs, beaten
- Olive oil for brushing

Instructions:

1. Preheat the oven to 400°F (200°C).

2. In a bowl, combine grated zucchini, whole wheat flour, Parmesan, garlic, oregano, salt, and pepper.

3. Stir in beaten eggs until well combined.

4. Drop spoonfuls onto a baking sheet, brush with olive oil.

5. Bake for 15-20 minutes or until golden brown.

Prep Time: 25 minutes

6. Roasted Red Pepper Hummus

Ingredients:

- 1 can (15 oz) chickpeas, drained and rinsed
- 2 roasted red peppers, peeled and chopped
- 1/4 cup tahini
- 2 tablespoons olive oil
- 1 clove garlic, minced
- Juice of 1 lemon
- Salt and cayenne pepper to taste
- Whole grain pita or veggie sticks for serving

Instructions:

1. In a food processor, blend chickpeas, roasted red peppers, tahini, olive oil, garlic, and lemon juice until smooth.

2. Season with salt and cayenne pepper. Adjust to taste.

3. Serve with whole grain pita or veggie sticks.

Prep Time: 15 minutes

7. Sweet Potato and Black Bean Quesadillas

Ingredients:

- 2 medium sweet potatoes, peeled and grated
- 1 can (15 oz) black beans, drained and rinsed
- 1 cup shredded cheddar cheese
- 1 teaspoon ground cumin
- 1/2 teaspoon chili powder
- Salt and pepper to taste
- Whole grain tortillas
- Salsa and Greek yogurt for serving

Instructions:

1. In a bowl, mix grated sweet potatoes, black beans, cheddar cheese, cumin, chili powder, salt, and pepper.

2. Divide the mixture evenly and place it on half of each tortilla.

3. Fold the tortillas in half and cook on a skillet until the cheese is melted and tortillas are golden.

4. Serve with salsa and Greek yogurt.

Prep Time: 30 minutes

8. Caprese Skewers with Balsamic Glaze

Ingredients:

- Cherry tomatoes
- Fresh mozzarella balls
- Fresh basil leaves
- Balsamic glaze
- Wooden skewers

Instructions:

1. Thread a cherry tomato, a fresh mozzarella ball, and a basil leaf onto each skewer.

2. Arrange on a serving platter.

3. Drizzle with balsamic glaze just before serving.

Prep Time: 15 minutes

9. Edamame and Mint Dip

Ingredients:

- 1 cup edamame, shelled and cooked
- 2 tablespoons fresh mint leaves

- 1 clove garlic
- Juice of 1 lime
- 2 tablespoons olive oil
- Salt and pepper to taste
- Whole grain crackers or veggie sticks for serving

Instructions:

1. In a food processor, blend edamame, mint, garlic, lime juice, and olive oil until smooth.

2. Season with salt and pepper. Adjust to taste.

3. Serve with whole grain crackers or veggie sticks

Prep Time: 15 minutes

10. Tomato Basil Bruschetta

Ingredients:

- 4 tomatoes, diced
- 1/4 cup fresh basil, chopped
- 2 cloves garlic, minced
- 2 tablespoons balsamic vinegar
- 2 tablespoons olive oil
- Salt and pepper to taste
- Whole grain baguette slices

Instructions:

1. In a bowl, combine tomatoes, basil, garlic, balsamic vinegar, and olive oil.

2. Season with salt and pepper. Mix well.

3. Toast the whole grain baguette slices and top with the tomato-basil mixture.

Prep Time: 20 minutes

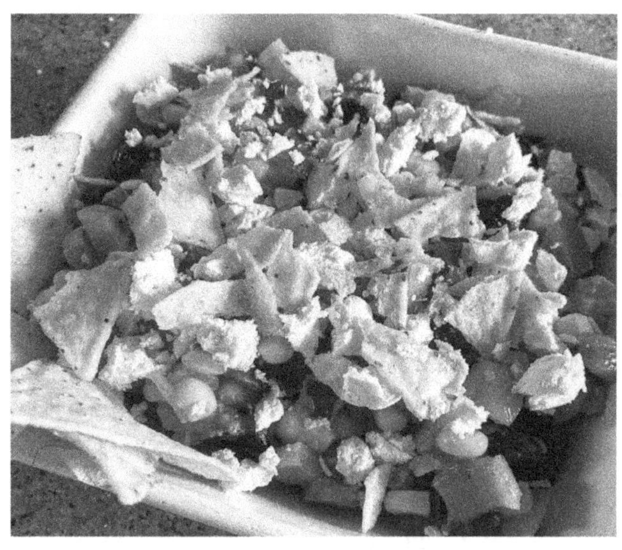

CHAPTER 4

Vibrant Salads

1. Rainbow Quinoa Salad

Ingredients:

- 1 cup cooked quinoa
- 1 cup cherry tomatoes, halved
- 1 cucumber, diced
- 1 bell pepper (any color), diced
- 1/2 red onion, finely chopped
- 1/4 cup feta cheese, crumbled
- 2 tablespoons olive oil
- Juice of 1 lemon
- Salt and pepper to taste
- Fresh parsley for garnish

Instructions:

1. In a large bowl, combine cooked quinoa, cherry tomatoes, cucumber, bell pepper, red onion, and feta cheese.

2. In a small bowl, whisk together olive oil, lemon juice, salt, and pepper.

3. Drizzle the dressing over the salad and toss gently.

4. Garnish with fresh parsley before serving.

Prep Time: 20 minutes

2. Chickpea and Roasted Vegetable Salad

Ingredients:

- 1 can (15 oz) chickpeas, drained and rinsed
- 1 zucchini, diced
- 1 eggplant, diced
- 1 red onion, sliced
- 1 bell pepper (any color), sliced
- 2 tablespoons olive oil
- 1 teaspoon cumin
- 1 teaspoon smoked paprika
- Salt and pepper to taste
- Mixed greens for the base
- Balsamic vinaigrette for dressing

Instructions:

1. Preheat the oven to 400°F (200°C).

2. Toss chickpeas, zucchini, eggplant, red onion, and bell pepper with olive oil, cumin, smoked paprika, salt, and pepper.

3. Roast in the oven for 25-30 minutes until vegetables are tender.

4. Arrange mixed greens on a serving plate, top with the roasted vegetable mixture, and drizzle with balsamic vinaigrette.

Prep Time: 35 minutes

3. Kale and Cranberry Power Salad

Ingredients:

- 4 cups kale, stems removed and chopped
- 1 cup cooked quinoa
- 1/2 cup dried cranberries
- 1/4 cup pumpkin seeds
- 1/4 cup feta cheese, crumbled
- 2 tablespoons olive oil
- Juice of 1 orange
- 1 tablespoon Dijon mustard
- Salt and pepper to taste

- Orange zest for garnish

Instructions:

1. In a large bowl, massage kale with olive oil until slightly softened.

2. Add cooked quinoa, dried cranberries, pumpkin seeds, and feta cheese.

3. In a small bowl, whisk together orange juice, Dijon mustard, salt, and pepper.

4. Drizzle the dressing over the salad and toss gently.

5. Garnish with orange zest before serving.

Prep Time: 20 minutes

4. Mediterranean Quinoa Salad

Ingredients:

- 1 cup cooked quinoa
- 1 cup cherry tomatoes, halved
- 1 cucumber, diced
- 1/2 red onion, finely chopped
- 1/2 cup Kalamata olives, sliced
- 1/2 cup crumbled feta cheese
- 3 tablespoons olive oil

- Juice of 1 lemon

- 1 teaspoon dried oregano

- Salt and pepper to taste

- Fresh mint for garnish

Instructions:

1. In a large bowl, combine cooked quinoa, cherry tomatoes, cucumber, red onion, olives, and feta cheese.

2. In a small bowl, whisk together olive oil, lemon juice, dried oregano, salt, and pepper.

3. Drizzle the dressing over the salad and toss gently.

4. Garnish with fresh mint before serving.

Prep Time: 20 minutes

5. Roasted Beet and Goat Cheese Salad

Ingredients:

- 3 medium beets, roasted and sliced

- 4 cups arugula

- 1/2 cup walnuts, toasted and chopped

- 1/4 cup goat cheese, crumbled

- 2 tablespoons balsamic vinegar
- 2 tablespoons olive oil
- 1 teaspoon honey
- Salt and pepper to taste

Instructions:

1. Preheat the oven to 400°F (200°C).

2. Wrap beets in foil and roast for 45-60 minutes until tender. Let them cool, peel, and slice.

3. In a large bowl, combine arugula, roasted beets, toasted walnuts, and goat cheese.

4. In a small bowl, whisk together balsamic vinegar, olive oil, honey, salt, and pepper.

5. Drizzle the dressing over the salad and toss gently before serving.

Prep Time: 1 hour (including roasting time)

6. Asian-Inspired Edamame Salad

Ingredients:

- 2 cups edamame, shelled and cooked
- 1 red bell pepper, julienned
- 1 carrot, julienned
- 1 cup red cabbage, thinly sliced

- 1/4 cup cilantro, chopped
- 3 tablespoons soy sauce
- 1 tablespoon sesame oil
- 1 tablespoon rice vinegar
- 1 teaspoon honey
- Sesame seeds for garnish

Instructions:

1. In a large bowl, combine edamame, red bell pepper, carrot, red cabbage, and cilantro.

2. In a small bowl, whisk together soy sauce, sesame oil, rice vinegar, and honey.

3. Drizzle the dressing over the salad and toss gently.

4. Garnish with sesame seeds before serving.

Prep Time: 15 minutes

7. Quinoa and Avocado Salad with Cilantro-Lime Dressing

Ingredients:

- 1 cup cooked quinoa
- 2 avocados, diced
- 1 cup cherry tomatoes, halved

- 1/4 cup red onion, finely chopped
- 1/4 cup fresh cilantro, chopped
- Juice of 2 limes
- 2 tablespoons olive oil
- Salt and pepper to taste
- Radish slices for garnish

Instructions:

1. In a large bowl, combine cooked quinoa, diced avocados, cherry tomatoes, red onion, and cilantro.

2. In a small bowl, whisk together lime juice, olive oil, salt, and pepper.

3. Drizzle the dressing over the salad and toss gently.

4. Garnish with radish slices before serving.

Prep Time: 20 minutes

8. Orange and Fennel Salad

Ingredients:

- 1 can (15 oz) chickpeas, drained and rinsed
- 1 zucchini, diced
- 1 eggplant, diced
- 1 red onion, sliced

- 1 bell pepper (any color), sliced

- 2 tablespoons olive oil

- 1 teaspoon cumin

- 1 teaspoon smoked paprika

- Salt and pepper to taste

- Mixed greens for the base

- Balsamic vinaigrette, thinly sliced

- 1/4 cup red onion, thinly sliced

- 1/4 cup sliced almonds, toasted

- 2 tablespoons extra virgin olive oil

- 1 tablespoon white balsamic vinegar

- Salt and pepper to taste

Instructions:

1. In a large bowl, combine mixed salad greens, orange segments, sliced fennel, red onion, and toasted almonds.

2. In a small bowl, whisk together olive oil, white balsamic vinegar, salt, and pepper.

3. Drizzle the dressing over the salad and toss gently before serving.

Prep Time: 15 minutes

9. Broccoli and Chickpea Salad

Ingredients:

- 2 cups broccoli florets, blanched
- 1 can (15 oz) chickpeas, drained and rinsed
- 1/2 cup cherry tomatoes, halved
- 1/4 cup red onion, finely chopped
- 1/4 cup feta cheese, crumbled
- 2 tablespoons lemon juice
- 2 tablespoons olive oil
- 1 teaspoon Dijon mustard
- Salt and pepper to taste
- Sunflower seeds for garnish

Instructions:

1. In a large bowl, combine blanched broccoli, chickpeas, cherry tomatoes, red onion, and feta cheese.

2. In a small bowl, whisk together lemon juice, olive oil, Dijon mustard, salt, and pepper.

3. Drizzle the dressing over the salad and toss gently.

4. Garnish with sunflower seeds before serving.

Prep Time: 20 minute

10. Spicy Mexican Black Bean Salad

Ingredients:

- 2 cans (15 oz each) black beans, drained and rinsed
- 1 cup corn kernels (fresh or frozen, thawed)
- 1 red bell pepper, diced
- 1/2 red onion, finely chopped
- 1 jalapeño, seeded and diced
- 1/4 cup fresh cilantro, chopped
- Juice of 2 limes
- 3 tablespoons olive oil
- 1 teaspoon cumin
- 1/2 teaspoon chili powder
- Salt and pepper to taste
- Avocado slices for garnish

Instructions:

1. In a large bowl, combine black beans, corn, red bell pepper, red onion, jalapeño, and cilantro.

2. In a small bowl, whisk together lime juice, olive oil, cumin, chili powder, salt, and pepper.

3. Drizzle the dressing over the salad and toss gently.

4. Garnish with avocado slices before serving.

Prep Time: 20 minutes

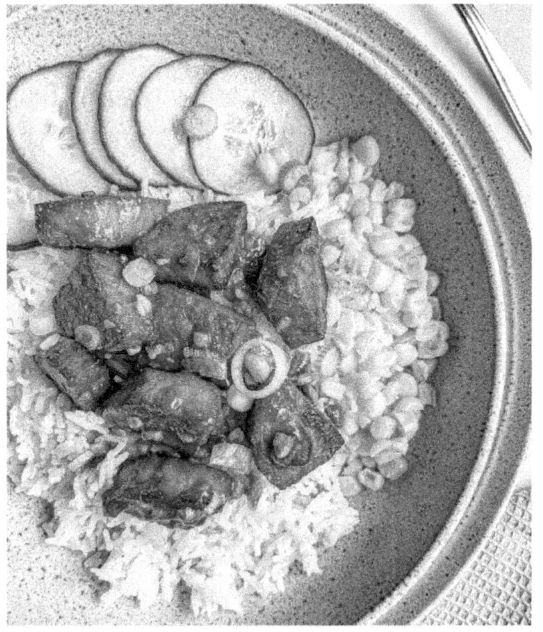

CHAPTER 5

Satisfying Main Courses

1. Lentil and Vegetable Stew

Ingredients:

- 1 cup dry green or brown lentils, rinsed
- 4 cups vegetable broth
- 1 onion, diced
- 2 carrots, chopped
- 2 celery stalks, chopped
- 3 cloves garlic, minced
- 1 can (14 oz) diced tomatoes
- 1 teaspoon cumin
- 1 teaspoon smoked paprika
- Salt and pepper to taste
- Fresh parsley for garnish

Instructions:

1. In a large pot, sauté onions, carrots, and celery until softened.

2. Add garlic, cumin, and smoked paprika; cook for another minute.

3. Stir in lentils, vegetable broth, and diced tomatoes.

4. Bring to a boil, then simmer until lentils are tender (about 25-30 minutes).

5. Season with salt and pepper. Garnish with fresh parsley before serving.

Prep Time: 40 minutes

2. Chickpea and Vegetable Stir-Fry

Ingredients:

- 2 cans (15 oz each) chickpeas, drained and rinsed
- 1 broccoli head, cut into florets
- 1 bell pepper (any color), sliced
- 1 zucchini, sliced
- 1 carrot, julienned
- 3 tablespoons soy sauce
- 1 tablespoon sesame oil
- 1 tablespoon maple syrup
- 1 teaspoon ginger, minced

- 2 cloves garlic, minced
- Brown rice or quinoa for serving

Instructions:

1. In a wok or large skillet, stir-fry chickpeas, broccoli, bell pepper, zucchini, and carrot until vegetables are tender-crisp.

2. In a small bowl, whisk together soy sauce, sesame oil, maple syrup, ginger, and garlic.

3. Pour the sauce over the stir-fry and toss until well coated.

4. Serve over brown rice or quinoa.

Prep Time: 25 minutes

3. Spinach and Mushroom Stuffed Bell Peppers

Ingredients:

- 4 bell peppers, halved and seeds removed
- 2 cups cooked quinoa
- 1 cup baby spinach, chopped
- 1 cup mushrooms, finely chopped
- 1 onion, finely chopped
- 2 cloves garlic, minced

- 1 can (15 oz) black beans, drained and rinsed
- 1 teaspoon cumin
- 1 teaspoon chili powder
- Salt and pepper to taste
- 1 cup shredded cheese (cheddar or your choice)

Instructions:

1. Preheat the oven to 375°F (190°C).

2. In a skillet, sauté onions, mushrooms, and garlic until softened.

3. In a large bowl, combine cooked quinoa, chopped spinach, sautéed vegetables, black beans, cumin, chili powder, salt, and pepper.

4. Stuff each bell pepper half with the quinoa mixture.

5. Sprinkle shredded cheese on top.

6. Bake for 25-30 minutes or until the peppers are tender.

Prep Time: 40 minutes

4. Sweet Potato and Black Bean Enchiladas

Ingredients:

- 2 large sweet potatoes, peeled and diced
- 1 can (15 oz) black beans, drained and rinsed
- 1 red onion, diced
- 1 bell pepper (any color), diced
- 1 teaspoon cumin
- 1 teaspoon chili powder
- 8 whole wheat tortillas
- 2 cups enchilada sauce
- 1 cup shredded cheese (cheddar or your choice)
- Fresh cilantro for garnish

Instructions:

1. Preheat the oven to 375°F (190°C).

2. Steam or roast sweet potatoes until tender.

3. In a bowl, mash sweet potatoes and mix with black beans, red onion, bell pepper, cumin, and chili powder.

4. Fill each tortilla with the sweet potato mixture and roll up.

5. Place the rolled tortillas in a baking dish, pour enchilada sauce over them, and sprinkle with shredded cheese.

6. Bake for 20-25 minutes or until the cheese is melted and bubbly.

7. Garnish with fresh cilantro before serving.

Prep Time: 45 minutes

5. Eggplant and Chickpea Curry

Ingredients:

- 1 large eggplant, diced
- 1 can (15 oz) chickpeas, drained and rinsed
- 1 onion, finely chopped
- 2 tomatoes, diced
- 3 cloves garlic, minced
- 1 tablespoon curry powder
- 1 teaspoon cumin
- 1 teaspoon coriander
- 1/2 teaspoon turmeric
- 1 can (14 oz) coconut milk

- Salt and pepper to taste
- Fresh cilantro for garnish
- Cooked brown rice for serving

Instructions:

1. In a large pot, sauté onions and garlic until softened.

2. Add diced eggplant, chickpeas, tomatoes, curry powder, cumin, coriander, and turmeric.

3. Stir in coconut milk and simmer until the eggplant is tender (about 20 minutes).

4. Season with salt and pepper. Garnish with fresh cilantro.

5. Serve over cooked brown rice.

Prep Time: 40 minutes

6. Butternut Squash and Sage Risotto

Ingredients:

- 2 cups butternut squash, diced
- 1 cup Arborio rice
- 1/2 cup dry white wine
- 4 cups vegetable broth, heated
- 1 onion, finely chopped

- 2 cloves garlic, minced
- 2 tablespoons olive oil
- 1/4 cup fresh sage, chopped
- 1/2 cup grated Parmesan cheese
- Salt and pepper to taste

Instructions:

1. In a skillet, sauté onions and garlic in olive oil until softened.

2. Add Arborio rice and cook until lightly toasted.

3. Pour in the white wine and cook until mostly absorbed.

4. Begin adding the vegetable broth, one ladle at a time, stirring frequently until the liquid is absorbed.

5. Add diced butternut squash and continue adding broth until the rice is creamy and cooked.

6. Stir in chopped sage, Parmesan cheese, salt, and pepper.

7. Serve warm.

Prep Time: 40 minutes

7. Quinoa and Black Bean Stuffed Peppers

Ingredients:

- 4 bell peppers, halved and seeds removed
- 1 cup quinoa, cooked
- 1 can (15 oz) black beans, drained and rinsed
- 1 cup corn kernels (fresh or frozen, thawed)
- 1 cup salsa
- 1 teaspoon cumin
- 1 teaspoon chili powder
- 1/2 cup shredded cheese (cheddar or your choice)
- Fresh cilantro for garnish

Instructions:

1. Preheat the oven to 375°F (190°C).

2. In a bowl, mix cooked quinoa, black beans, corn, salsa, cumin, and chili powder.

3. Fill each bell pepper half with the quinoa mixture.

4. Sprinkle shredded cheese on top.

5. Bake for 20-25 minutes or until the peppers are tender.

6. Garnish with fresh cilantro before serving.

Prep Time: 35 minutes

8. Mushroom and Spinach Stuffed Portobello Mushrooms

Ingredients:

- 4 large portobello mushrooms, stems removed
- 2 cups baby spinach, chopped
- 1 cup mushrooms, finely chopped
- 1 onion, finely chopped
- 2 cloves garlic, minced
- 1/2 cup breadcrumbs
- 1/4 cup grated Parmesan cheese
- 2 tablespoons olive oil
- Salt and pepper to taste
- Fresh parsley for garnish

Instructions:

1. Preheat the oven to 375°F (190°C).

2. In a skillet, sauté onions, garlic, and chopped mushrooms until softened.

3. Add chopped spinach and cook until wilted.

4. In a bowl, mix sautéed mixture with breadcrumbs and Parmesan cheese.

5. Fill each portobello mushroom cap with the stuffing.

6. Drizzle with olive oil and bake for 20-25 minutes.

7. Garnish with fresh parsley before serving.

Prep Time: 35 minutes

9. Zucchini Noodles with Pesto and Cherry Tomatoes

Ingredients:

- 4 medium zucchinis, spiralized into noodles
- 1 cup cherry tomatoes, halved
- 1/2 cup pine nuts, toasted
- 1/2 cup fresh basil leaves
- 1/4 cup grated Parmesan cheese
- 2 cloves garlic
- 1/2 cup extra virgin olive oil

- Salt and pepper to taste

Instructions:

1. In a food processor, blend basil, pine nuts, Parmesan, garlic, salt, and pepper.

2. While blending, gradually add olive oil until the pesto is smooth.

3. In a large skillet, sauté zucchini noodles until just tender.

4. Toss zucchini noodles with cherry tomatoes and pesto.

5. Serve warm.

Prep Time: 25 minutes

10. Quinoa and Vegetable Stuffed Acorn Squash

Ingredients:

- 2 acorn squash, halved and seeds removed
- 1 cup quinoa, cooked
- 1 cup kale, chopped
- 1 cup chickpeas, cooked
- 1/2 cup dried cranberries
- 1/4 cup pecans, chopped

- 1/4 cup feta cheese, crumbled

- 2 tablespoons olive oil

- 1 tablespoon balsamic vinegar

- Salt and pepper to taste

Instructions:

1. Preheat the oven to 375°F (190°C).

2. Place acorn squash halves on a baking sheet, cut side up.

3. In a bowl, mix cooked quinoa, chopped kale, chickpeas, dried cranberries, pecans, and feta cheese.

4. Stuff each acorn squash half with the quinoa mixture.

5. Drizzle with olive oil and balsamic vinegar.

6. Bake for 30-35 minutes or until the squash is tender.

Prep Time: 45 minutes

CHAPTER 6

Wholesome Side Dishes

1. Roasted Brussels Sprouts with Balsamic Glaze

Ingredients:

- 1 lb Brussels sprouts, trimmed and halved
- 2 tablespoons olive oil
- Salt and pepper to taste
- 2 tablespoons balsamic glaze

Instructions:

1. Preheat the oven to 400°F (200°C).

2. Toss Brussels sprouts with olive oil, salt, and pepper.

3. Roast for 20-25 minutes or until golden brown.

4. Drizzle with balsamic glaze before serving.

Prep Time: 30 minutes

2. Lemon Garlic Quinoa

Ingredients:

- 1 cup quinoa, rinsed
- 2 cups vegetable broth
- 2 tablespoons olive oil
- 2 cloves garlic, minced
- Zest and juice of 1 lemon
- Salt and pepper to taste
- Fresh parsley for garnish

Instructions:

1. In a saucepan, bring vegetable broth to a boil.

2. Add quinoa, reduce heat, cover, and simmer until cooked (about 15 minutes).

3. In a skillet, sauté garlic in olive oil until fragrant.

4. Fluff quinoa with a fork and stir in the garlic, lemon zest, lemon juice, salt, and pepper.

5. Garnish with fresh parsley before serving.

Prep Time: 20 minutes

3. Grilled Asparagus with Parmesan

Ingredients:

- 1 lb asparagus, trimmed
- 2 tablespoons olive oil
- Salt and pepper to taste

- 1/4 cup grated Parmesan cheese
- Lemon wedges for serving

Instructions:

1. Preheat the grill or grill pan over medium heat.

2. Toss asparagus with olive oil, salt, and pepper.

3. Grill for 5-7 minutes, turning occasionally, until tender.

4. Sprinkle with Parmesan cheese and serve with lemon wedges.

Prep Time: 15 minutes

4. Mediterranean Quinoa Salad

Ingredients:

- 1 cup cooked quinoa
- 1 cucumber, diced
- 1 cup cherry tomatoes, halved
- 1/2 red onion, finely chopped
- 1/2 cup Kalamata olives, sliced
- 1/4 cup crumbled feta cheese
- 3 tablespoons olive oil
- Juice of 1 lemon
- 1 teaspoon dried oregano

- Salt and pepper to taste
- Fresh mint for garnish

Instructions:

1. In a bowl, combine cooked quinoa, cucumber, cherry tomatoes, red onion, olives, and feta cheese.

2. In a small bowl, whisk together olive oil, lemon juice, dried oregano, salt, and pepper.

3. Drizzle the dressing over the salad and toss gently.

4. Garnish with fresh mint before serving.

Prep Time: 20 minutes

5. Garlic Herb Roasted Sweet Potatoes

Ingredients:

- 3 large sweet potatoes, peeled and diced
- 3 tablespoons olive oil
- 3 cloves garlic, minced
- 1 teaspoon dried thyme
- 1 teaspoon dried rosemary
- Salt and pepper to taste
- Fresh parsley for garnish

Instructions:

1. Preheat the oven to 400°F (200°C).

2. In a bowl, toss sweet potatoes with olive oil, garlic, thyme, rosemary, salt, and pepper.

3. Spread on a baking sheet and roast for 25-30 minutes or until golden and tender.

4. Garnish with fresh parsley before serving.

Prep Time: 35 minutes

6. Quinoa and Black Bean Salad

Ingredients:

- 1 cup cooked quinoa
- 1 can (15 oz) black beans, drained and rinsed
- 1 cup corn kernels (fresh or frozen, thawed)
- 1/2 red onion, finely chopped
- 1/4 cup cilantro, chopped
- Juice of 2 limes
- 3 tablespoons olive oil
- Salt and pepper to taste
- Avocado slices for garnish

Instructions:

1. In a bowl, combine cooked quinoa, black beans, corn, red onion, cilantro, lime juice, and olive oil.

2. Season with salt and pepper. Toss gently.

3. Refrigerate for at least 30 minutes before serving.

4. Garnish with avocado slices.

Prep Time: 20 minutes

7. Baked Parmesan Zucchini Fries

Ingredients:

- 4 medium zucchinis, cut into fries
- 1 cup breadcrumbs
- 1/2 cup grated Parmesan cheese
- 1 teaspoon garlic powder
- 1/2 teaspoon dried oregano
- Salt and pepper to taste
- 2 eggs, beaten
- Marinara sauce for dipping

Instructions:

1. Preheat the oven to 425°F (220°C).

2. In a bowl, combine breadcrumbs, Parmesan cheese, garlic powder, oregano, salt, and pepper.

3. Dip zucchini fries into beaten eggs, then coat with the breadcrumb mixture.

4. Place on a baking sheet and bake for 20-25 minutes or until golden brown.

5. Serve with marinara sauce for dipping.

Prep Time: 30 minutes

8. Cabbage and Apple Slaw

Ingredients:

- 1/2 head green cabbage, thinly sliced
- 2 apples, julienned
- 1/2 cup Greek yogurt
- 2 tablespoons Dijon mustard
- 1 tablespoon honey
- 1 tablespoon apple cider vinegar
- Salt and pepper to taste
- Chopped walnuts for garnish

Instructions:

1. In a large bowl, combine sliced cabbage and julienned apples.

2. In a small bowl, whisk together Greek yogurt, Dijon mustard, honey, apple cider vinegar, salt, and pepper.

3. Pour the dressing over the cabbage and apples, tossing to coat.

4. Garnish with chopped walnuts before serving.

Prep Time: 15 minutes

9. Lemon Herb Quinoa Pilaf

Ingredients:

- 1 cup quinoa, rinsed
- 2 cups vegetable broth
- 2 tablespoons olive oil
- Zest and juice of 1 lemon
- 1 teaspoon dried thyme
- 1 teaspoon dried parsley
- Salt and pepper to taste
- Chopped chives for garnish

Instructions:

1. In a saucepan, bring vegetable broth to a boil.

2. Add quinoa, reduce heat, cover, and simmer until cooked (about 15 minutes).

3. In a skillet, heat olive oil and sauté lemon zest, lemon juice, thyme, parsley, salt, and pepper.

4. Fluff quinoa with a fork and toss with the lemon herb mixture.

5. Garnish with chopped chives before serving.

Prep Time: 20 minutes

10. Tomato Basil Farro Risotto

Ingredients:

- 1 cup farro
- 4 cups vegetable broth, heated
- 2 tablespoons olive oil
- 1 onion, finely chopped
- 2 cloves garlic, minced
- 1 can (14 oz) diced tomatoes
- 1/2 cup fresh basil, chopped
- 1/2 cup grated Parmesan cheese
- Salt and pepper to taste

Instructions:

1. In a skillet, sauté onions and garlic in olive oil until softened.

2. Add farro and cook until lightly toasted.

3. Begin adding the heated vegetable broth, one ladle at a time, stirring frequently until the liquid is absorbed.

4. Stir in diced tomatoes and continue adding broth until the farro is creamy and cooked.

5. Stir in chopped basil, Parmesan cheese, salt, and pepper.

6. Serve warm.

Prep Time: 40 minutes

CHAPTER 7

Flavorful Snacks

1. Roasted Chickpeas with Smoky Paprika

Ingredients:

- 2 cans (15 oz each) chickpeas, drained and rinsed
- 2 tablespoons olive oil
- 1 teaspoon smoked paprika
- 1/2 teaspoon cumin
- 1/2 teaspoon garlic powder
- Salt and pepper to taste

Instructions:

1. Preheat the oven to 400°F (200°C).

2. Pat the chickpeas dry and toss with olive oil, smoked paprika, cumin, garlic powder, salt, and pepper.

3. Spread them on a baking sheet and bake for 25-30 minutes or until crispy.

4. Allow to cool before serving.

Prep Time: 35 minutes

2. Guacamole with Veggie Sticks

Ingredients:

- 3 ripe avocados, mashed
- 1 tomato, diced
- 1/4 cup red onion, finely chopped
- 1/4 cup cilantro, chopped
- Juice of 1 lime
- Salt and pepper to taste
- Carrot and cucumber sticks for dipping

Instructions:

1. In a bowl, combine mashed avocados, diced tomato, red onion, cilantro, lime juice, salt, and pepper.

2. Mix well and serve with carrot and cucumber sticks for dipping.

Prep Time: 15 minutes

3. Spicy Edamame

Ingredients:

- 2 cups edamame, steamed
- 1 tablespoon olive oil
- 1 teaspoon chili powder
- 1/2 teaspoon smoked paprika
- 1/2 teaspoon garlic powder
- Salt to taste

Instructions:

1. In a bowl, toss steamed edamame with olive oil, chili powder, smoked paprika, garlic powder, and salt.

2. Serve warm or at room temperature.

Prep Time: 15 minutes

4. Mediterranean Hummus Plate

Ingredients:

1 cup hummus

1/2 cup cherry tomatoes, halved

1/2 cucumber, sliced

1/4 cup Kalamata olives

1/4 cup feta cheese, crumbled

1 tablespoon olive oil

Pita bread or whole grain crackers for serving

Instructions:

1. Spread hummus on a serving plate.

2. Arrange cherry tomatoes, cucumber slices, Kalamata olives, and crumbled feta on top.

3. Drizzle with olive oil and serve with pita bread or whole grain crackers.

Prep Time: 10 minutes

5. Stuffed Mini Bell Peppers

Ingredients:

- 12 mini bell peppers, halved and seeds removed
- 1 cup black beans, canned and drained
- 1/2 cup corn kernels (fresh or frozen, thawed)
- 1/4 cup red onion, finely chopped
- 1/4 cup cilantro, chopped
- Juice of 1 lime
- Salt and pepper to taste

Instructions:

1. In a bowl, mix black beans, corn, red onion, cilantro, lime juice, salt, and pepper.

2. Stuff each mini bell pepper half with the mixture.

3. Serve chilled.

Prep Time: 20 minutes

6. Kale Chips

Ingredients:

- 1 bunch kale, stems removed and torn into bite-sized pieces
- 2 tablespoons olive oil
- 1 teaspoon nutritional yeast
- 1/2 teaspoon garlic powder
- Salt to taste

Instructions:

1. Preheat the oven to 300°F (150°C).

2. In a bowl, toss kale with olive oil, nutritional yeast, garlic powder, and salt.

3. Spread on a baking sheet and bake for 20-25 minutes or until crisp.

4. Allow to cool before serving.

Prep Time: 30 minutes

7. Mango Salsa with Whole Grain Tortilla Chips

Ingredients:

- 2 mangoes, diced
- 1/2 red onion, finely chopped
- 1 jalapeño, seeded and finely chopped
- 1/4 cup fresh cilantro, chopped
- Juice of 2 limes
- Salt and pepper to taste
- Whole grain tortilla chips for dipping

Instructions:

1. In a bowl, combine diced mangoes, red onion, jalapeño, cilantro, lime juice, salt, and pepper.

2. Mix well and serve with whole grain tortilla chips.

Prep Time: 15 minutes

8. Quinoa Stuffed Mushrooms

Ingredients:

- 12 large mushrooms, stems removed
- 1 cup cooked quinoa
- 1/2 cup sun-dried tomatoes, chopped

- 1/4 cup pine nuts, toasted
- 1/4 cup fresh basil, chopped
- 2 tablespoons olive oil
- 1 clove garlic, minced
- Salt and pepper to taste

Instructions:

1. Preheat the oven to 375°F (190°C).

2. In a bowl, mix cooked quinoa, sun-dried tomatoes, pine nuts, basil, olive oil, garlic, salt, and pepper.

3. Stuff each mushroom cap with the quinoa mixture.

4. Bake for 15-20 minutes or until mushrooms are tender.

Prep Time: 30 minutes

9. Avocado and Black Bean Salsa

Ingredients:

- 2 avocados, diced
- 1 can (15 oz) black beans, drained and rinsed
- 1/2 red onion, finely chopped

- 1/4 cup fresh cilantro, chopped
- Juice of 1 lime
- Salt and pepper to taste
- Tortilla chips for serving

Instructions:

1. In a bowl, combine diced avocados, black beans, red onion, cilantro, lime juice, salt, and pepper.

2. Mix well and serve with tortilla chips.

Prep Time: 15 minutes

10. Greek Yogurt and Berry Parfait

Ingredients:

- 1 cup Greek yogurt
- 1 cup mixed berries (strawberries, blueberries, raspberries)
- 1/4 cup granola
- 1 tablespoon honey

Instructions:

1. In a glass or bowl, layer Greek yogurt, mixed berries, and granola.

2. Drizzle with honey before serving.

Prep Time: 10 minutes

CHAPTER 8

Delectable Desserts

1. Chocolate Avocado Mousse

Ingredients:

- 2 ripe avocados
- 1/4 cup cocoa powder
- 1/4 cup maple syrup
- 1 teaspoon vanilla extract
- Pinch of salt
- Fresh berries for garnish

Instructions:

1. In a blender or food processor, combine avocados, cocoa powder, maple syrup, vanilla extract, and a pinch of salt.

2. Blend until smooth and creamy.

3. Chill in the refrigerator for at least 1 hour before serving.

4. Garnish with fresh berries before serving.

Prep Time: 15 minutes

2. Chia Seed Pudding with Mixed Berries

Ingredients:

- 1/4 cup chia seeds
- 1 cup almond milk (or any plant-based milk)
- 1 tablespoon maple syrup
- 1/2 teaspoon vanilla extract
- Mixed berries for topping

Instructions:

1. In a bowl, whisk together chia seeds, almond milk, maple syrup, and vanilla extract.

2. Refrigerate for at least 2 hours or overnight, stirring occasionally.

3. Serve topped with mixed berries.

Prep Time: 5 minutes (+ chilling time)

3. Oat and Banana Cookies

Ingredients:

- 2 ripe bananas, mashed
- 1 cup rolled oats
- 1/4 cup raisins

- 1/4 cup chopped nuts (walnuts, almonds, or your choice)
- 1 teaspoon vanilla extract
- 1/2 teaspoon cinnamon

Instructions:

1. Preheat the oven to 350°F (180°C).

2. In a bowl, mix mashed bananas, rolled oats, raisins, chopped nuts, vanilla extract, and cinnamon.

3. Drop spoonfuls of the mixture onto a baking sheet.

4. Bake for 15-20 minutes or until golden brown.

5. Allow to cool before serving.

Prep Time: 10 minutes

4. Berry and Almond Crisp

Ingredients:

- 4 cups mixed berries (strawberries, blueberries, raspberries)
- 1/4 cup maple syrup
- 1 teaspoon lemon juice
- 1 cup rolled oats
- 1/2 cup almond flour

- 1/4 cup sliced almonds
- 1/4 cup coconut oil, melted
- 1/4 cup maple syrup
- Vanilla ice cream or yogurt for serving

Instructions:

1. Preheat the oven to 350°F (180°C).

2. In a bowl, toss mixed berries with maple syrup and lemon juice. Transfer to a baking dish.

3. In another bowl, mix rolled oats, almond flour, sliced almonds, melted coconut oil, and maple syrup.

4. Crumble the oat mixture over the berries.

5. Bake for 30-35 minutes or until the topping is golden brown.

6. Serve warm with vanilla ice cream or yogurt.

Prep Time: 20 minutes

5. Fig and Walnut Energy Bites

Ingredients:

- 1 cup dried figs, stemmed
- 1 cup walnuts
- 1/4 cup rolled oats

- 1 tablespoon chia seeds
- 1 teaspoon vanilla extract
- Pinch of salt
- Shredded coconut for coating (optional)

Instructions:

1. In a food processor, combine dried figs, walnuts, rolled oats, chia seeds, vanilla extract, and a pinch of salt.

2. Pulse until the mixture comes together.

3. Roll into small balls and coat with shredded coconut if desired.

4. Refrigerate for at least 30 minutes before serving.

Prep Time: 15 minutes

6. Apple Cinnamon Baked Oatmeal

Ingredients:

- 2 cups rolled oats
- 1 teaspoon baking powder
- 1 teaspoon cinnamon
- 1/4 teaspoon nutmeg
- 2 cups almond milk
- 1/4 cup maple syrup

- 2 apples, peeled and diced
- 1/4 cup chopped nuts (pecans or almonds)
- Greek yogurt for serving

Instructions:

1. Preheat the oven to 375°F (190°C).

2. In a bowl, mix rolled oats, baking powder, cinnamon, and nutmeg.

3. Add almond milk, maple syrup, diced apples, and chopped nuts. Stir well.

4. Transfer to a baking dish and bake for 30-35 minutes or until set.

5. Serve warm with a dollop of Greek yogurt.

Prep Time: 15 minutes

7. Pumpkin and Pecan Muffins

Ingredients:

- 1 cup canned pumpkin
- 1/2 cup maple syrup
- 1/4 cup coconut oil, melted
- 2 flax eggs (2 tablespoons ground flaxseeds + 6 tablespoons water)
- 1 teaspoon vanilla extract

- 1 1/2 cups whole wheat flour
- 1 teaspoon baking powder
- 1/2 teaspoon baking soda
- 1/2 teaspoon cinnamon
- 1/4 teaspoon nutmeg
- Pinch of salt
- 1/2 cup chopped pecans

Instructions:

1. Preheat the oven to 350°F (180°C) and line a muffin tin with liners.

2. In a bowl, whisk together pumpkin, maple syrup, melted coconut oil, flax eggs, and vanilla extract.

3. In another bowl, whisk together whole wheat flour, baking powder, baking soda, cinnamon, nutmeg, and a pinch of salt.

4. Add the wet ingredients to the dry ingredients and mix until just combined.

5. Fold in chopped pecans.

6. Divide the batter into muffin cups and bake for 18-20 minutes or until a toothpick comes out clean.

7. Allow to cool before serving.

Prep Time: 20 minutes

8. Date and Walnut Bars

Ingredients:

- 1 cup pitted dates
- 1 cup walnuts
- 1/2 cup rolled oats
- 1/4 cup almond butter
- 1 teaspoon vanilla extract
- Pinch of salt
- Dark chocolate drizzle (optional)

Instructions:

1. In a food processor, combine pitted dates, walnuts, rolled oats, almond butter, vanilla extract, and a pinch of salt.

2. Pulse until the mixture forms a sticky dough.

3. Press the mixture into a lined baking dish.

4. If desired, drizzle with melted dark chocolate.

5. Refrigerate for at least 1 hour before cutting into bars.

Prep Time: 15 minutes

9. Coconut Mango Chia Pudding

Ingredients:

- 1/4 cup chia seeds
- 1 cup coconut milk
- 1 tablespoon maple syrup
- 1/2 teaspoon vanilla extract
- 1 ripe mango, diced
- Shredded coconut for topping

Instructions:

1. In a bowl, whisk together chia seeds, coconut milk, maple syrup, and vanilla extract.

2. Refrigerate for at least 2 hours or overnight, stirring occasionally.

3. Layer with diced mango and top with shredded coconut before serving.

Prep Time: 5 minutes (+ chilling time)

10. Blueberry Almond Crumble Bars

Ingredients:

- 2 cups rolled oats
- 1 cup almond flour
- 1/2 cup coconut oil, melted
- 1/4 cup maple syrup
- 1/2 teaspoon baking soda

- 1/4 teaspoon salt
- 1 1/2 cups blueberries
- 1/4 cup sliced almonds

Instructions:

1. Preheat the oven to 350°F (180°C) and line a baking dish with parchment paper.

2. In a bowl, mix rolled oats, almond flour, melted coconut oil, maple syrup, baking soda, and salt.

3. Press half of the mixture into the bottom of the prepared dish.

4. Sprinkle blueberries evenly over the crust.

5. Crumble the remaining oat mixture over the blueberries.

6. Top with sliced almonds.

7. Bake for 25-30 minutes or until golden brown.

8. Allow to cool before cutting into bars.

Prep Time: 20 minutes

CHAPTER 9

Beverages and Smoothies

1. Green Fiber Boost Smoothie

Ingredients:

- 1 cup spinach leaves
- 1/2 cucumber, peeled and sliced
- 1/2 avocado
- 1/2 banana
- 1 tablespoon chia seeds
- 1 cup almond milk
- Ice cubes (optional)

Instructions:

1. In a blender, combine spinach, cucumber, avocado, banana, chia seeds, and almond milk.

2. Blend until smooth.

3. Add ice cubes if desired and blend again.

4. Pour into a glass and enjoy!

Prep Time: 5 minutes

2. Berry and Flaxseed Smoothie

Ingredients:

- 1 cup mixed berries (strawberries, blueberries, raspberries)
- 1 tablespoon flaxseeds
- 1/2 cup Greek yogurt
- 1 cup almond milk
- 1 tablespoon honey
- Ice cubes (optional)

Instructions:

1. In a blender, combine mixed berries, flaxseeds, Greek yogurt, almond milk, and honey.

2. Blend until smooth.

3. Add ice cubes if desired and blend again.

4. Pour into a glass and enjoy!

Prep Time: 5 minutes

3. Tropical Fiber Delight Smoothie

Ingredients:

- 1/2 cup pineapple chunks
- 1/2 cup mango chunks
- 1/2 banana

- 1 tablespoon hemp seeds
- 1 cup coconut water
- Ice cubes (optional)

Instructions:

1. In a blender, combine pineapple, mango, banana, hemp seeds, and coconut water.

2. Blend until smooth.

3. Add ice cubes if desired and blend again.

4. Pour into a glass and enjoy!

Prep Time: 5 minutes

4. Kale and Pineapple Detox Smoothie

Ingredients:

- 1 cup kale leaves, stems removed
- 1/2 cup pineapple chunks
- 1/2 green apple, cored and sliced
- 1 tablespoon chia seeds
- 1 cup coconut water
- Ice cubes (optional)

Instructions:

1. In a blender, combine kale, pineapple, green apple, chia seeds, and coconut water.

2. Blend until smooth.

3. Add ice cubes if desired and blend again.

4. Pour into a glass and enjoy!

Prep Time: 5 minutes

5. Blueberry and Oatmeal Smoothie

Ingredients:

- 1/2 cup blueberries
- 1/4 cup rolled oats
- 1/2 banana
- 1 tablespoon almond butter
- 1 cup almond milk
- Ice cubes (optional)

Instructions:

1. In a blender, combine blueberries, rolled oats, banana, almond butter, and almond milk.

2. Blend until smooth.

3. Add ice cubes if desired and blend again.

4. Pour into a glass and enjoy!

Prep Time: 5 minutes

6. Citrus and Carrot Energizer Juice

Ingredients:

- 2 oranges, peeled and segmented
- 1 carrot, peeled and sliced
- 1/2 lemon, juiced
- 1/2-inch piece of ginger, grated
- 1 cup water
- Ice cubes (optional)

Instructions:

1. In a blender, combine orange segments, carrot slices, lemon juice, grated ginger, and water.

2. Blend until smooth.

3. Strain the juice using a fine mesh sieve.

4. Add ice cubes if desired and stir.

5. Pour into a glass and enjoy!

Prep Time: 5 minutes

7. Beet and Berry Antioxidant Smoothie

Ingredients:

- 1/2 cup cooked beets, chopped

- 1/2 cup mixed berries (blueberries, raspberries)
- 1/2 cup Greek yogurt
- 1 tablespoon ground flaxseeds
- 1 cup almond milk
- Ice cubes (optional)

Instructions:

1. In a blender, combine cooked beets, mixed berries, Greek yogurt, flaxseeds, and almond milk.

2. Blend until smooth.

3. Add ice cubes if desired and blend again.

4. Pour into a glass and enjoy!

Prep Time: 5 minutes

8. Spinach and Banana Protein Smoothie

Ingredients:

- 1 cup spinach leaves
- 1/2 banana
- 1/2 cup plain Greek yogurt
- 1 scoop vanilla protein powder
- 1 cup almond milk

- Ice cubes (optional)

Instructions:

1. In a blender, combine spinach, banana, Greek yogurt, protein powder, and almond milk.

2. Blend until smooth.

3. Add ice cubes if desired and blend again.

4. Pour into a glass and enjoy!

Prep Time: 5 minutes

9. Pumpkin Pie Smoothie

Ingredients:

- 1/2 cup canned pumpkin
- 1/2 banana
- 1/2 teaspoon pumpkin pie spice
- 1 tablespoon chia seeds
- 1 cup almond milk
- Ice cubes (optional)

Instructions:

1. In a blender, combine canned pumpkin, banana, pumpkin pie spice, chia seeds, and almond milk.

2. Blend until smooth.

3. Add ice cubes if desired and blend again.

4. Pour into a glass and enjoy!

Prep Time: 5 minutes

10.   Chocolate   Almond   Butter Smoothie

Ingredients:

- 1 tablespoon almond butter
- 1 tablespoon cocoa powder
- 1/2 banana
- 1 tablespoon chia seeds
- 1 cup almond milk
- Ice cubes (optional)

Instructions:

1. In a blender, combine almond butter, cocoa powder, banana, chia seeds, and almond milk.

2. Blend until smooth.

3. Add ice cubes if desired and blend again.

4. Pour into a glass and enjoy!

Prep Time: 5 minutes

CHAPTER 10

Meal Planning and Tips

Tips for Grocery Shopping

To ensure you have a range of nutrient-rich meals, grocery shopping for a high-fiber vegetarian diet takes careful planning. Here are some grocery shopping ideas to help you live a high-fiber vegetarian lifestyle:

1. Make a grocery list:

- Plan your meals for the week and make a shopping list based on the recipes you've chosen. This allows you to stay focused and avoid making impulse purchases.

2. Include a Wide Range of Whole Grains:

- Whole grains such as quinoa, brown rice, oats, barley, and whole wheat products are ideal. These grains are high in fiber and contain critical nutrients.

3. Fill Up on Legumes:

- Fiber and protein are abundant in beans, lentils, and chickpeas. To have convenient options for quick dinners, use both canned and dried kinds.

4. Eat a Variety of Fruits and Vegetables:

- Include a variety of bright fruits and veggies in your shopping cart. These contain a wide range of vitamins, minerals, and antioxidants. Fresh, frozen, and canned (no added sugar) foods are all viable possibilities.

5. Select High-Fiber Vegetables:

- Fiber-rich vegetables include broccoli, Brussels sprouts, kale, spinach, carrots, and cauliflower. These adaptable ingredients can be used in salads, stir-fries, and side dishes.

6. Invest in Nuts and Seeds:

- Fiber, healthy fats, and protein are abundant in almonds, walnuts, chia seeds, flaxseeds, and sunflower seeds. For a nutritional boost, mix them into cereals, yogurt, or salads.

7. Investigate Dairy and Nondairy Alternatives:

- Choose low-fat dairy products or plant-based alternatives such as almond milk, soy milk, or oat milk. These can be good calcium and vitamin D sources.

8. Examine Food Labels:

- Pay close attention to food labels to find high-fiber options. Look for products that contain whole grains, legumes, and are minimally processed.

9. Plant-based protein sources should be included:

- Tofu, tempeh, seitan, and plant-based protein substitutes are good sources of protein and can be utilized in a number of cuisines.

10. Don't Forget Healthy Fats:

- Avocados, olives, and oils such as olive oil and avocado oil are wonderful sources of healthful fats. Use them in moderation for cooking or as toppings.

11. Buy in Bulk:

- Purchasing goods like grains, beans, and nuts in bulk can save money and reduce packaging waste. Ensure proper storage to maintain freshness.

12. Check the Perimeter of the Store:

- Whole, minimally processed items including fruits, vegetables, whole grains, and fresh produce are frequently located around the perimeter of the grocery store. Focus on these areas for healthier choices.

13. Consider Frozen Fruits and Vegetables:

- Frozen fruits and vegetables are often just as healthy as fresh ones and have a longer shelf life. They can be convenient for adding to smoothies or as side dishes.

14. Minimize Processed Foods:

- Limit the intake of processed foods, as they may have extra sweets, harmful fats, and less nutrients. Stick to whole, natural foods wherever possible.

15. Keep Hydrated:

- Keep water and other nutritious beverages on your shopping list. Staying hydrated is essential for overall health.

You can prepare a well-balanced and fiber-rich vegetarian shopping list that meets your nutritional needs by following these guidelines.

Weekly Meal Plans

Day 1:

Breakfast:

- Greek yogurt parfait with mixed berries, chia seeds, and a drizzle of honey
- Whole grain toast with avocado slices

Lunch:

- Quinoa and black bean salad with diced tomatoes, cucumber, and a lime-cilantro dressing

Dinner:

- Lentil and vegetable curry served over brown rice

- Steamed broccoli on the side

Snack:

- Apple slices with almond butter

Day 2:

Breakfast:

- Oatmeal topped with sliced bananas, chopped nuts, and a sprinkle of cinnamon
- Orange slices on the side

Lunch:

- Spinach and feta stuffed bell peppers
- Whole wheat pita bread

Dinner:

- Roasted sweet potato and chickpea Buddha bowl with tahini dressing

Snack:

- Carrot sticks with hummus

Day 3:

Breakfast:

- Smoothie with spinach, frozen berries, banana, chia seeds, and almond milk

Lunch:

- Quinoa-stuffed portobello mushrooms with a side of mixed green salad

Dinner:

- Whole grain spaghetti with homemade tomato and vegetable sauce
- Grilled zucchini and eggplant on the side

Snack:

- Handful of mixed nuts

Day 4:

Breakfast:

- Whole grain toast with smashed avocado and cherry tomatoes
- Freshly squeezed orange juice

Lunch:

- Chickpea and vegetable stir-fry with brown rice

Dinner:

- Baked falafel wraps with whole wheat tortillas, shredded lettuce, tomatoes, and tzatziki sauce

Snack:

- Greek yogurt with a handful of granola

Day 5:

Breakfast:

- Chia seed pudding made with almond milk, topped with sliced strawberries and kiwi

Lunch:

- Lentil and vegetable soup with a side of whole grain crackers

Dinner:

- Quinoa and black bean stuffed bell peppers with a side of salsa

Snack:

- Sliced cucumber with guacamole

Day 6:

Breakfast:

- Banana and blueberry smoothie with oats and a scoop of almond butter

Lunch:

- Whole wheat wrap with hummus, shredded carrots, cucumber, and spinach

Dinner:

- Grilled vegetable and tofu kebabs with quinoa
- Side of mixed green salad with balsamic vinaigrette

Snack:

- Popcorn seasoned with nutritional yeast

Day 7:

Breakfast:

- Overnight oats with almond milk, topped with mixed berries and sliced almonds

Lunch:

- Mediterranean quinoa salad with cherry tomatoes, Kalamata olives, feta cheese, and a lemon vinaigrette

Dinner:

- Eggplant and chickpea curry with basmati rice
- Steamed asparagus on the side

Snack:

- Sliced apple with a sprinkle of cinnamon

CONCLUSION

We've discovered a world of tastes, colors, and nourishment while investigating a high-fiber vegetarian diet. This cookbook is more than just a compilation of recipes; it is also a guide to a healthier and more lively way of living. Let us enjoy the richness that comes from nature's bounty as we wrap up this gastronomic adventure: fiber-rich fruits, veggies, whole grains, and legumes.

Embracing this high-fiber vegetarian lifestyle is about cultivating a beneficial impact on our well-being, not just what's on the plate. We are not only pleasing our taste buds but also our body when we choose fiber-rich foods. The advantages go beyond the kitchen and include higher energy, better digestion, and a sense of vibrancy in our daily life.

May this cookbook inspire you to cook wonderful, nutritious meals that will nourish your body and bring joy to your table. Let the vivid salads, robust soups, and filling main courses attest to the nutritional value of a high-fiber vegetarian diet. Here's to savoring every bite, appreciating the path of good health, and exploring the limitless possibilities of a plant-powered, fiber-filled life. Enjoy your cooking and eating!

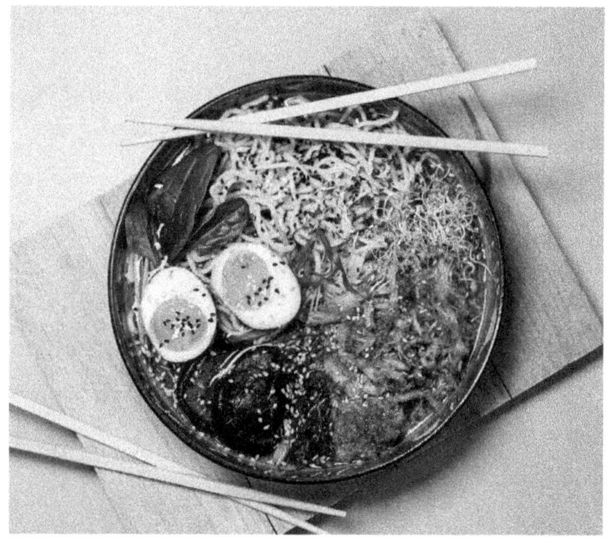

www.ingramcontent.com/pod-product-compliance
Lightning Source LLC
Chambersburg PA
CBHW071606270726
48661CB00019B/1610